VEGAN DIET COOKBOOK FOR ATHLETES

Everything You Need to Know about Veganism, plus Delicious Plant-Based Recipes with High-Protein Foods Appropriate for Bodybuilders' Athletic Performance

Willy Stone

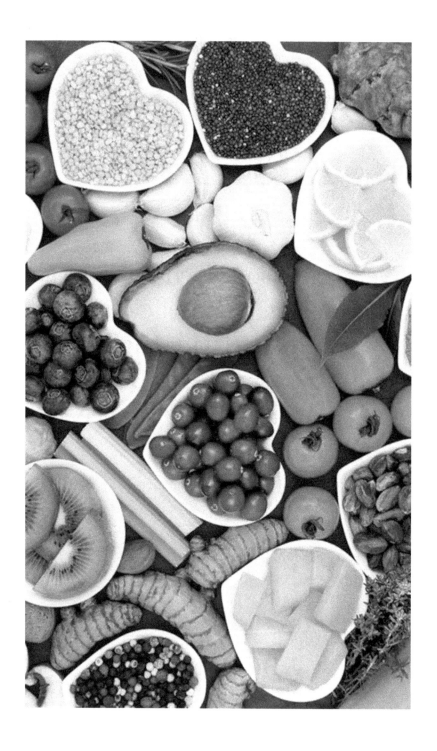

Table of Contents

WHY VEGAN DIET FOR ATHLETES?

Can you become vegan and expect to maintain or even improve upon your athletic performance? DEFINITELY! Not only is it possible, but it also happens all the time. Some examples of which are six-time ironman champion Ruth Heidrich, professional and Olympic skating sensation Charlene Wong Williams, U.S. national team synchronized swimmer Kim Wurzel, power-lifting champion Pat Reeves, or any one of the thousands of other successful vegan and near-vegan athletes. The key to fueling peak performance is getting the right balance of energy and nutrients. If you are an athlete, whether a starter or a professional, you'll want to maximize your potential with the best nutrition possible.

FUELING THE VEGAN ATHLETE

The energy needs of vegan athletes vary with body size, weight, composition, metabolism, gender, age, and the amount and type of physical activity performed. Physical activity increases energy needs and can also increase basal metabolic rate (BMR) by up to 30%. (BMR accounts for about 60–75% of total energy needs). Exercise can lead to increased energy output for up to 24 hours after the exercise is stopped. This is a very minor increase, but it can make a difference in the long term. Also, eating a whole foods vegan diet may increase energy requirements by up to 10–15% due to reduced overall digestibility of high-fiber whole foods.

For individuals exercising casually a few times a week, energy needs increase only slightly, if at all. For those training more intensely several times a week, energy needs can be as high as 3,000–6,000 calories a day or more.

WHAT IS A VEGAN DIET

Veganism is one type of vegetarian diet. Exclusions for those who are vegan include any meat, dairy products, eggs, and any other ingredients that are derived from animals. A growing number of people who follow a vegan diet also do not eat any type of food that has been processed using any kind of animal products, including certain types of wines and white sugar that has been refined. The actual term "vegan" can either refer to the diet itself or a person who has adopted this style of eating.

To those who are not familiar with Veganism, this is the most common question that is asked. Many people have visions of a plate of salad night after night for the rest of their lives. In reality, a vegan diet is quite diverse. It includes fruits, vegetables, legumes, beans, and all grains. Think of the infinite combination of delicious meals that can be made from these ingredients! There are also vegan options for most of the popular dishes people enjoy eating. Some common examples include vegan mayonnaise, vegan cheese, vegan ice cream, vegan hot dogs, vegan pizza, and tons of others. Veganism is steadily gaining in popularity these days as the awareness about leading environment-friendly lifestyles is increasing. Along with its popularity, the general misconceptions about this diet are rising as well. All these widespread misconceptions have managed to trigger a somewhat restrictive and negative attitude toward veganism. These misconceptions are the only reason why a lot of people hesitate before transitioning to veganism. Going vegan might seem like a fad, but it is the best way to lead an environmentally conscious life.

This book contains proven steps and strategies on how to harness the power of a vegan diet. It will discuss what a vegan diet is, how to become vegan, the most popular reasons to become vegan, famous athletes who are proudly vegan, and also talk about some of the supplements that are available for vegans.

If you would like to try the vegan lifestyle, you need to get it right from the start. Many people have given it a go but never really got to grips with it. To be honest, it is never easy because there isn't really a great deal of support around. But just like anything worth doing, stick at it and the results will come.

For those athletes who have successfully adopted the vegan ways, they have noticed some great benefits. One of those is that the body recovers quicker between training sessions. As you can imagine, if the athlete has a faster recovery, they can train more often and see quicker improvements. It's not the increased amount of training that is the best thing; it's the faster recovery that allows for the additional training. That's important.

Veganism is the new buzzword all over the world, with health fanatics steadily moving to a vegan diet for purported health advantages and the ethics about the treatment of animals. It has not only got the general population to take to this new form of living but also many athletes, sportsmen, and bodybuilders. However, to get the same amount of proteins from the plant-based diet as from an animal diet is quite severe. Hence, it requires a measured form of eating the right proteins and in proper quantities to extract maximum protein. This is of especially paramount importance to athletes and bodybuilders as a lot of energy and calories are burned during physical activity and, thus need to be replaced with good proteins to get the desired effects. Vegan bodybuilding for beginners can be tough but not impossible. It is undoubtedly a herculean task to get proteins from a plant-based diet, but there are ways and means to

"Anyone interested in bodybuilding requires large doses of protein to develop muscles. Reaching the protein goals while removing dairy and meat from the diet might not sound **plausible; however, a vegan diet doesn't need** *to hold you back. You can attain all the protein your body needs without ever worrying about compromising the health of your muscles or your body in general."*

This book is about using a vegan diet as fuel to live a more athletic lifestyle. You need to eat daily, so why not eat fibrous, nutritious, and plant-load your meals? I genuinely believe that with the information contained in this book, together with a keen interest in athletic living, you will see that it is not difficult to eat a vegan diet and that anyone can take a vegan diet at any level.

Now, if you are ready to learn more, then let us get started without further ado!

BENEFITS ASSOCIATED WITH VEGAN DIETS

Before we get started talking about how you can live on a vegan diet as an athlete, let's talk about the **WHY**. Why abandon meat-based meals in favor of being a vegan?

<u>Risk Factors Reduced By a Vegan Diet:</u>

Blood Cholesterol Level

It is estimated that for every 1% increase in blood cholesterol, heart disease risk increases by 2–3%. The most important dietary factors that raise blood cholesterol are saturated fat, cholesterol, and trans-fatty acids. Of all dietary groups, vegans have the lowest intakes of saturated fat, trans-fatty acids, and cholesterol. The most powerful cholesterol-lowering agents are soluble fiber, plant protein (especially soy protein), polyunsaturated fats, and phytochemicals, all of which are found exclusively or primarily in plant foods. It comes as no surprise that vegans have the lowest total and LDL cholesterol levels of all dietary groups, including Lacto-Ovo vegetarians and fish-eaters. In 5 studies from 1987–1999, average blood cholesterol of vegans ranged from 3.5 mmol/l (135 mg/dl) to 4.3 mmol/l (165 mg/dl), compared with 4.6 mmol/l (177 mg/dl) to 5.3 mmol/l (205 mg/dl) for nonvegetarians.

Oxidation of LDL Cholesterol

When LDL cholesterol becomes oxidized by free radicals, the product is highly damaging to blood vessels, inducing plaque formation. The susceptibility of LDL cholesterol to oxidation depends on both the levels of LDL cholesterol present and the presence of antioxidants such as vitamin E, carotenoids, vitamin C, flavonoids, and polyphenolic compounds. Also, high intakes of heme iron may increase LDL oxidation. (Heme iron is found only in meat, fish, and poultry.) Antioxidants come primarily from plant foods, so concentrations of these protective substances are typically higher in vegan diets than in nonvegetarian diets. Recent studies showed vegans to have higher blood levels of antioxidants and lower levels of lipid peroxidation than nonvegetarians.

Hypertension (high blood pressure)

Both coronary artery disease and stroke are increased by high blood pressure. While vegan and vegetarian populations have slightly lower blood pressures than nonvegetarians (5–10 mm Hg less), rates of hypertension are lower still, (only one-third to one-half those of nonvegetarians). The healthier bodyweight of vegans and vegetarians appears to be an important contributing factor. Other aspects of diet that may control blood pressure are higher fiber; higher potassium, magnesium, and phytochemical intakes; lower total and saturated fat consumption; and possibly reduced sodium intakes. (Vegans may not consume less sodium with high intakes of convenience foods.)

Obesity and High Waist-to-Hip Ratio

The risk of heart disease and hypertension are both associated with excessive body weight. Compared with Lacto-Ovo vegetarians and nonvegetarians, vegans are leaner and have lower waist-to-hip ratios. It is thought that low obesity rates are related to these characteristics of vegan diets: high fiber content (improves satiety), lower fat content (reduces caloric density), and higher glucagon secretion. (Glucagon increases blood glucose concentration, promotes appetite control, and increases fat oxidation.)

Blood Clotting Tendency

Most serious cardiovascular events (heart attacks, strokes, etc.) begin with the formation of a blood clot. Blood clots form and dissolve in blood all the time and generally do no harm. However, when injuries to blood vessels occur, this balance is disrupted, increasing the tendency for blood platelets to stick together (platelet aggregation). This is the initial step in clot formation. Once a clot is formed, it may attach to an artery wall or travel through the blood vessels, with the potential of becoming lodged and blocking blood flow. When blood flow to the heart is blocked, a heart attack occurs; when it occurs in the brain, the result is a stroke.

It has long been hypothesized that blood clotting tendencies would be decreased in vegetarians, and more so in vegans, due to a favorable ratio of saturated fat (which causes platelets to aggregate) compared to polyunsaturated fats. However, the few studies done have failed to support this theory. A possible explanation is that low vegan intakes of omega-3 fatty acids, which are about half the intakes of nonvegetarians, result in decreased production of potent hormone-like substances that reduce platelet aggregation. Li and coworkers, 1999, concluded that vegetarians, especially vegans, might be advised to increase their dietary intake of omega-3 fatty acids to reduce platelet aggregation.

Homocysteine Levels

Homocysteine is an amino acid produced by the body during the breakdown of methionine, a sulfur-containing essential amino acid that is concentrated in animal foods. There is strong evidence that elevated homocysteine is an independent risk factor for heart disease and may increase the risk of heart attack or stroke by two to three times. Research has failed to show a relationship between methionine intake and homocysteine levels but is centered more on intakes of three B vitamins that help us get rid of this damaging by-product. Blood levels of homocysteine are determined largely by folate, vitamins B12, and B6. Initially, researchers expected vegetarians and vegans to have low levels of homocysteine because they consume less methionine and almost twice as much folate as nonvegetarians. Instead, studies show average homocysteine levels of vegans to be either similar to or higher than nonvegetarians. Two studies (by Mezzano and by Mann, both 1999) found significantly higher homocysteine levels in vegetarians compared to meat-eaters, with vegans having the highest levels. Though vegan intakes of folate and B6 amounts are generally good, vegans may have reduced vitamin B12 status, increasing the risk for elevated homocysteine. Vitamin B12 is involved in the conversion of homocysteine back to methionine. With insufficient B12, conversion appears to be slowed, and homocysteine levels rise. On the other hand, one would expect vegan diets to reduce homocysteine levels if all three B vitamins are abundantly supplied.

Overall Risk for Heart Disease and

Vegans have a reduced risk for heart disease and stroke due to their high-fiber, low-saturated fat, cholesterol-free, phytochemical-rich diets. They have lower total and LDL cholesterol levels, lower blood pressure, less obesity, better waist/hip ratios, and lower levels of certain blood clotting factors. However, vegans appear to have higher platelet aggregation factors and may have higher homocysteine levels, which could, at least partly, counteract the benefits. The message is crystal clear:

"The vegan diet has tremendous potential for reducing heart disease risk."

<u>For full benefit:</u>

    • Ensure adequate intake of vitamin B12. (Use a supplement and/or B12-fortified foods.)

    • Ensure sufficient intake of omega-3 fatty acids and improve the balance of essential fatty acids. (For more on this, see Chapter 4.)

Vegan Diets in the Treatment of Cardiovascular Disease

Vegan and near-vegan diets have proven highly effective in treating cardiovascular diseases as shown in the result of multiple studies. Mediterranean-style diets are among the most protective diets against heart disease. Though not exclusively vegetarian, these are centered around relatively unprocessed plant foods, including nuts, seeds, olive oil, and avocados. In the Lyon Heart Study, by the end of two years on the Mediterranean diet patients had an *<u>unprecedented 76% lower risk of dying of a heart attack or stroke</u>* when compared with patients on a "prudent Western-type diet." Mediterranean diets are higher in monounsaturated fat and omega-3 fatty acids, and lower in omega-6 fatty acids than vegan diets. It is reasonable to assume that a vegan "Mediterranean-style" diet, constructed to avoid B12 shortages and to ensure sufficient omega-3 fatty acids, could produce even more impressive results. Such a diet would actually be lower in saturated fat and cholesterol and higher in fiber than traditional Mediterranean diets.

Vegans and Cancer...what we know

In light of the findings to date on specific food components and cancer, one would expect that the vegan diet would afford the greatest protection of all. While it appears very promising, the research that looks specifically at vegan diets is too limited to draw conclusions at this point.
In 1999 Key analyzed data from five prospective studies of mortality in vegetarians and nonvegetarians. While cancer mortality in vegans is assessed separately, the small population of vegans (753) relative to Lacto-

Ovo vegetarians (23,265) and nonvegetarians (42,276) makes the findings merely suggestive. The two largest prospective studies to date looking at the mortality of vegetarians were the Seventh-day Adventist (SDA) Mortality Study (comparing vegetarian Adventists with nonvegetarians in the general population) and the Adventist Health Study (comparing vegetarian and nonvegetarian Adventists). Pertinent findings from these studies are given.

Diabetes

Diabetes is the seventh leading cause of death in the U.S. and an important risk factor for heart disease, stroke, kidney disease, blindness, and leg and foot amputations. There are two types of diabetes:

• Type 1 (insulin-dependent diabetes mellitus or IDDM)—a lack of insulin production by the pancreas • Type 2 (noninsulin-dependent diabetes mellitus—NIDDM)—insulin resistance (pancreas produces insulin but the body is unable to use it efficiently)

Type 1 diabetes accounts for only about 10% of all cases. There are considerable global differences in Type 1 diabetes, and several observations have linked these differences to milk consumption. While some research indicates a pattern of increased diabetes with greater milk consumption, the pattern is not entirely consistent. A recent study by Elliot (1999) found that while total milk protein consumption did not consistently correlate with diabetes incidence, the consumption of specific milk proteins (beta-casein A + B) did. Different breeds of cows produce varying amounts of beta-casein A + B. These proteins produce a peptide called beta-casomorphin-7, which has immune-suppressing activity. While further research is warranted to determine the proportion of Type 1 diabetes caused by these milk proteins, we can expect that Type 1 diabetes would be less common among those who are raised as vegans without milk protein intake.

Type 2 diabetes is a disease that is seen with a frequency that varies tremendously across population groups, from virtually zero to as much as 50%. Approximately 80% of those suffering from Type 2 diabetes are overweight. Excess body weight is the single most important risk factor for Type 2 diabetes, especially for those who carry their weight in their upper body (apple shape), rather than hips and thighs (pear shape). The risk of diabetes is approximately doubled for those who are moderately overweight, tripled for those with frank obesity. For Type 2 diabetes, the most effective treatment is weight loss.

Incidence of Diabetes in Vegans and Vegetarians

Worldwide, the lowest frequency of Type 2 diabetes is with populations eating near-vegan diets. Whether this is due strictly to lower body weight is not yet clear. Some convincing evidence exists that very-high-fiber diets may, in themselves, be protective. When populations such as these adopt a high-fat, low-fiber North American-style diet, diabetes risk quickly escalates. If they revert to their original diet, the incidence of diabetes is once again reduced.

For Western vegetarians, evidence comes from a large study of Seventh-day Adventists (Snowdon, 1985). As yet no similar studies are looking at the incidence of diabetes in Western vegan populations; however, there are several reasons that vegans may be at reduced risk:

- less obesity

- lower intakes of saturated fat (may increase insulin secretion, potentially leading to insulin insensitivity*)

- much higher intakes of fiber, especially soluble fiber (improves blood glucose response)

- higher intakes of magnesium in well-designed vegan diets (insufficient magnesium may lead to insulin resistance)

- higher intakes of unrefined foods (whole grains, legumes, vegetables, nuts, seeds) with a low glycemic index.

Studies using low-fat vegan, vegetarian, or near-vegetarian diets for the treatment of cardiovascular disease have resulted in marked improvements in blood glucose control and reduced requirements for hypoglycemic medications.

Bone health

Vegan diets offer great and amazing advantages where bone health is concerned. However, vegans can expect to enjoy this excellent bone health throughout life by following the Vegan Food Guide and getting plenty of weight-bearing exercises, some of them in the sun. Whether one relies on the whole, calcium-rich plant foods and sunlight, or vegan products that are fortified with calcium and vitamin D, achieving excellent bone health can be accomplished with relative ease.

MAIN VEGAN FOOD CATEGORIES

What Are the Four Vegan Food Groups?

While there exist different types of vegan diets, they typically are always built from the same core principle, the exclusion of animal products - egg, meats, fish, honey, etc - as a result, vegans must work to balance their diets to ensure they receive adequate minerals and vitamins from their food. Aside from the daily eating of each of the four vegan food groups equally every day, there exist purely vegan supplements for iron, vitamin B12, and other nutrients and you should speak with your health care professional about them.

Fruit:

A vegan diet has a diverse and large variety of fruits available which while diverse are amazingly useful and should be eaten alongside every meal of the day: berries, citrus fruits, tree fruits, melons, vine fruits, and tropical fruits. Eating fruits along with your daily diet provides your body with folate, potassium, and vitamin C, amongst other minerals and vitamins.

Vitamin C promotes healing, Potassium helps in maintaining healthy blood pressure, and folate assists with the production of red blood cells.

Diversify your fruit intake by taking a variety of fruits including; oranges, tangerines, grapefruit, watermelon, apples, cantaloupe, grapes, peaches, bananas, strawberries, blueberries, mango, papaya, and kiwis.

Both frozen and fresh go well in salads and makes for delicious snacks. A fruit salad might also serve as a delicious and healthful dessert option.

Vegetables

With the absolute abundance variety of vegetables available, everybody is sure to find a few that suit their tastes. Cruciferous vegetables - broccoli, cauliflower, sprouts, brussels sprouts, kale and, cabbage - are nutrient-filled choices.

Leafy greens - arugula, chard, and butter lettuce are excellent for variety and creates the perfect base for both fruit and vegetable salads. Yams, eggplants, and potatoes go well with almost all types of seasoning and are filling enough and can serve as a main course at dinner or lunch.

Tomatoes and peppers, while technically fruits, usually fall in this category as well. Eating diets high in vegetables provides numerous benefits.

They are full of nutrients including dietary fiber which helps reduce overall risks of diseases and cholesterol levels as well as vitamin A which does miracles for eye health.

Whole Grains

Wheat, oats, brown rice, amaranth, quinoa, buckwheat, and barley are examples of whole grains to incorporate into your diet from sources including bread, pasta, cereals, and granolas. Whole grains exponentially expand the diversity of a vegan diet - pasta on which to serve tomato sauce pancakes to serve berries, oats to bring bulk to that green smoothie, quinoa as the base for steamed vegetables, or whole-grain bread used in making a grilled veggie sandwich.

Make your baked goods using whole grains; using egg replacements and other vegan adjustments to ensure you meet your dietary restrictions. Whole grains are great sources of vitamins including B vitamins which help keep your nervous system and entire metabolism functioning properly.

Legumes

Legumes - including chickpeas, soybeans, lentils, kidney beans, peas, and white beans - are excellent sources of protein in a vegan diet. They are so versatile: Cooked beans can be used as - a base for stews and soups, a bed for vegetables, a dip for vegetables, a thickener for sauces, a base for brownies, a meat patty substitute, it can even be a simple side dish. Soy products such as tempeh, soy milk, and tofu are excellent substitutes for eggs, meat, and dairy. Legumes, apart from providing proteins also provide fiber which does wonders in ensuring your digestive tract continues functioning properly.

Nuts and seeds, while not technically a part of the legume category are excellent sources of fats and protein - eat them as a snack or sprinkle them on cereals and salads. Consuming seeds and nuts reduces your risk of heart disease; however, ensure you select unsalted varieties and taking care to keep your sodium intake in check.

What to Eat

Here's a quick list of the foods that you should eat more of when you're on a plant-based diet program:

• Fruits – Berries, citrus fruits, apples, bananas, grapes, avocados, melons, dates, cantaloupe, apricots, cranberries, coconut, figs, guava, plums, kiwi, papaya, pears, pomelo, watermelon.

• Vegetables – Beetroot, broccoli, cauliflower, kale, carrots, potatoes, tomatoes, asparagus, red bell peppers, onions, garlic, ginger, zucchini, spinach, sweet potatoes, butternut squash, green beans.

• Legumes – Lentils, peas, chickpeas, kidney beans, black beans, navy beans, pinto beans, peanuts.

• Nuts – Almonds, walnuts, pistachios, hazelnuts, Brazilian nuts, cashews, pecans, macadamia.

- Seeds – Pumpkin seeds, chia seeds, flaxseeds, sunflower seeds, hemp seeds.

- Healthy oils – Olive oil, vegetable oil, avocado oil, flaxseed oil.

- Whole grains – Oats, brown rice, barley, quinoa, whole wheat bread, rye, buckwheat, spelled, cornmeal.

- Plant-based milk – Almond milk, soy milk, coconut milk, oat milk, rice milk, hemp milk.

- Seasonings, herbs, and spices – Salt, pepper, basil, rosemary, thyme, oregano, paprika, cumin, cinnamon.

- Beverages – Water, fresh fruit juices, smoothies, vegetable shakes.

What to Avoid

As for the foods to avoid, here's a list of those that you should avoid as much as possible:

- Meat – Beef, pork, lamb
- Seafood – Fish, shells, crabs, lobsters
- Poultry – Chicken, turkey, duck
- Dairy – Milk, butter, mayo, yogurt, cheese
- Other animal products – Eggs
- Processed foods
- Sugary treats
- Refined white carbohydrates
- High-sodium, high-fat food products
- Soda
- Alcohol

Tips to ensure success!

To help make sure that you achieve success with this diet program, take note of the following tips:

Write down your menu – Having a weekly menu eliminates the guesswork on what to prepare, and at the same time, helps you make use of your time more efficiently. When you're running late and don't know what to prepare for lunch or dinner, it's a lot easier to get tempted to go back to your old eating habits.

Focus on dishes that you love – The great thing about the plant-based diet is not as strict as other diet plans. And because it's versatile, you can focus on consuming dishes that you actually enjoy so that the transition will not feel too much like a chore.

Don't be too hard on yourself – Like any other diet program, the plant-based meal prep takes time and effort. If you are not patient enough, you will not achieve the results that you want.

Keep in mind that it's not something that can be achieved overnight.

BREAKFAST/ENERGY CHARGE

01. Fruity Granola

PREP: 15 MINUTES • COOK TIME: 45 MINUTES • TOTAL:60 MINUTES SERVES: 5

Ingredients

2 cups rolled oats

¾ cup whole-grain flour

1 tablespoon ground cinnamon

1 teaspoon ground ginger (optional)

½ cup sunflower seeds, or walnuts, chopped

½ cup almonds, chopped

½ cup pumpkin seeds

½ cup unsweetened shredded coconut

1¼ cups pure fruit juice (cranberry, apple, or something similar)

½ cup raisins, or dried cranberries

½ cup goji berries (optional)

Directions

Preparing the Ingredients.

Preheat the oven to 350°F.

Mix together the oats, flour, cinnamon, ginger, sunflower seeds, almonds, pumpkin seeds, and coconut in a large bowl.

Sprinkle the juice over the mixture, and stir until it's just moistened. You might need a bit more or a bit less liquid, depending on how much your oats and flour absorb.

Spread the granola on a large baking sheet (the more spread out it is the better), and put it in the oven. After about 15 minutes, use a spatula to turn the granola so that the middle gets dried out. Let the granola bake until it's as crunchy as you want it, about 30 minutes more.

Take the granola out of the oven and stir in the raisins and goji berries (if using). Store leftovers in an airtight container for up to 2 weeks.

Serve with non-dairy milk and fresh fruit, use as a topper for morning porridge or a smoothie bowl to add a bit of crunch, or make a granola parfait by layering with non-dairy yogurt or puréed banana.

Per Serving (½ cup) Calories: 398; Protein: 11g; Total fat: 25g; Carbohydrates: 39g; Fiber: 8g

02. **Pumpkin Steel-Cut Oats**

PREP: 2 MINUTES • COOK TIME: 35
MINUTES • TOTAL:37 MINUTES
SERVES: 4

Ingredients

3 cups water

1 cup steel-cut oats

½ cup canned pumpkin purée

¼ cup pumpkin seeds (pepitas)

2 tablespoons maple syrup

Pinch salt

Directions

Preparing the Ingredients.

In a large saucepan, bring the water to a boil.
Add the oats, stir, and reduce the heat to low.
Simmer until the oats are soft, 20 to 30
minutes, continuing to stir occasionally.

Stir in the pumpkin purée and continue
cooking on low for 3 to 5 minutes longer. Stir
in the pumpkin seeds and maple syrup, and
season with the salt.

Divide the oatmeal into 4 single-serving
containers. Let cool before sealing the lids.

Place the containers in the refrigerator for up to 5 days.

Per Serving: Calories:121; Protein: 4g; Total fat: 5g; Carbohydrates: 17g; Fiber: 2g

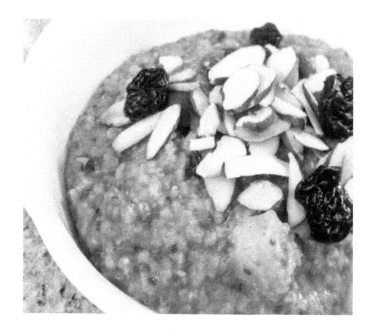

03. Chocolate Quinoa Breakfast Bowl

PREP: 5 MINUTES • COOK TIME: 30 MINUTES • TOTAL:35 MINUTES SERVES: 2

Ingredients

1 cup quinoa

1 teaspoon ground cinnamon

1 cup non-dairy milk

1 cup water

1 large banana

2 to 3 tablespoons unsweetened cocoa powder, or carob

1 to 2 tablespoons almond butter, or other nut or seed butter

1 tablespoon ground flaxseed, or chia or hemp seeds

2 tablespoons walnuts

¼ cup raspberries

Directions

Preparing the Ingredients.

Put the quinoa, cinnamon, milk, and water in a medium pot. Bring to a boil over high heat, then turn down low and simmer, covered, for 25 to 30 minutes.

While the quinoa is simmering, purée or mash the banana in a medium bowl and stir in the cocoa powder, almond butter, and flaxseed.

To serve, spoon 1 cup cooked quinoa into a bowl, top with half the pudding and half the walnuts and raspberries.

Per Serving: Calories: 392; Protein: 12g; Total fat: 19g; Saturated fat: 1g; Carbohydrates: 49g; Fiber: 10g

04

Muesli and Berries Bowl

PREP: 10 MINUTES • COOK TIME: 0
MINUTES • TOTAL:10 MINUTES
SERVES: 5

Ingredients

FOR THE MUESLI

1 cup rolled oats

1 cup spelled flakes, or quinoa flakes, or more rolled oats

2 cups puffed cereal

¼ cup sunflower seeds

¼ cup almonds

¼ cup raisins

¼ cup dried cranberries

¼ cup chopped dried figs

¼ cup unsweetened shredded coconut

¼ cup non-dairy chocolate chips

1 to 3 teaspoons ground cinnamon

FOR THE BOWL

½ cup non-dairy milk, or unsweetened applesauce

¾ cup muesli

½ cup berries

Directions

Preparing the Ingredients.

Put the muesli ingredients in a container or bag and shake.

Combine the muesli and bowl ingredients in a bowl or to-go container.

Substitutions: Try chopped Brazil nuts, peanuts, dried cranberries, dried blueberries, dried mango, or whatever inspires you. Ginger and cardamom are interesting flavors if you want to branch out on spices.

Per Serving: Calories: 441; Protein: 10g; Total fat: 20g; Carbohydrates: 63g; Fiber: 13g.

05

Cinnamon and Spice

PREP: 10 MINUTES • OVERNIGHT TO SOAK
SERVES: 5

Ingredients

2 ½ cups old-fashioned rolled oats

5 tablespoons pumpkin seeds (pepitas)

5 tablespoons chopped pecans

5 cups unsweetened plant-based milk

2½ teaspoons maple syrup or agave syrup

½ to 1 teaspoon salt

½ to 1 teaspoon ground cinnamon

½ to 1 teaspoon ground ginger

Fresh fruit (optional)

Directions

Preparing the Ingredients.

Line up 5 wide-mouth pint jars. In each jar, combine ½ cup of oats, 1 tablespoon of pumpkin seeds, 1 tablespoon of pecans, 1 cup of plant-based milk, ½ teaspoon of maple syrup, 1 pinch of salt, 1 pinch of cinnamon, and 1 pinch of ginger.

Stir the ingredients in each jar. Close the jars tightly with lids. To serve, top with fresh fruit (if using). Place the airtight jars in the refrigerator at least overnight before eating and for up to 5 days.

Per Serving: Calories:177; Protein: 6g; Total fat: 9g; Carbohydrates: 19g; Fiber: 4g.

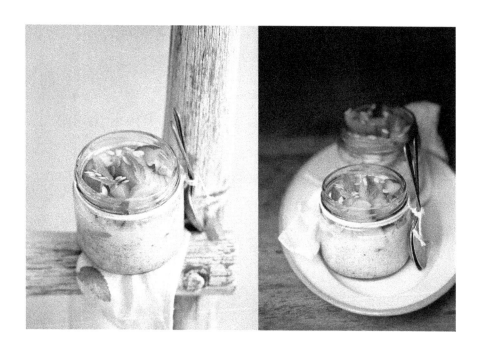

06. Baked Banana French Toast with Raspberry Syrup

PREP: 10 MINUTES • COOK TIME: 30 MINUTES • TOTAL: 40 MINUTES SERVES: 8 SLICES

Ingredients

FOR THE FRENCH TOAST

1 banana

1 cup coconut milk

1 teaspoon pure vanilla extract

¼ teaspoon ground nutmeg

½ teaspoon ground cinnamon

1½ teaspoons arrowroot powder

Pinch sea salt

8 slices whole-grain bread

FOR THE RASPBERRY SYRUP

1 cup fresh or frozen raspberries, or other berries

2 tablespoons water, or pure fruit juice

1 to 2 tablespoons maple syrup, or coconut sugar (optional)

Directions

Preparing the Ingredients.

Preheat the oven to 350°F.

In a shallow bowl, purée or mash the banana well. Mix in the coconut milk, vanilla, nutmeg, cinnamon, arrowroot, and salt.

Dip the slices of bread in the banana mixture, and then lay them out in a 13-by-9-inch baking dish.

They should cover the bottom of the dish and can overlap a bit but shouldn't be stacked on top of each other. Pour any leftover banana mixture over the bread, and put the dish in the oven.

Bake about 30 minutes, or until the tops are lightly browned.

Serve topped with raspberry syrup.

To Make the Raspberry Syrup

Heat the raspberries in a small pot with the water and the maple syrup (if using) on medium heat.

Leave to simmer, stirring occasionally, and breaking up the berries, for 15 to 20 minutes, until the liquid has reduced.

The leftover raspberry syrup makes a great topping for simple oatmeal as a quick and delicious breakfast, or as a drizzle on top of whole-grain toast smeared with natural peanut butter.

Per Serving: Calories: 166; Protein: 5g; Total fat: 7g; Saturated fat: 1g; Carbohydrates: 23g;

07. **Sunshine Muffins**

PREP: 15 MINUTES • COOK TIME: 30 MINUTES • TOTAL: 45 MINUTES SERVES: 6

Ingredients

1 teaspoon coconut oil, for greasing muffin tins (optional)

2 tablespoons almond butter, or sunflower seed butter

¼ cup non-dairy milk

1 orange, peeled

1 carrot, coarsely chopped

2 tablespoons chopped dried apricots, or other dried fruit

3 tablespoons molasses

2 tablespoons ground flaxseed

1 teaspoon apple cider vinegar

1 teaspoon pure vanilla extract

½ teaspoon ground cinnamon

½ teaspoon ground ginger (optional)

¼ teaspoon ground nutmeg (optional)

¼ teaspoon allspice (optional)

¾ cup rolled oats or whole-grain flour

1 teaspoon baking powder

½ teaspoon baking soda

MIX-INS (OPTIONAL)

½ cup rolled oats

2 tablespoons raisins, or other chopped dried fruit

2 tablespoons sunflower seeds

Directions

Preparing the Ingredients.

Preheat the oven to 350°F.

Prepare a 6-cup muffin tin by rubbing the insides of the cups with coconut oil or using silicone or paper muffin cups.

Purée the nut butter, milk, orange, carrot, apricots, molasses, flaxseed, vinegar, vanilla, cinnamon, ginger, nutmeg, and allspice in a food processor or blender until somewhat smooth.

Grind the oats in a clean coffee grinder until they're the consistency of flour (or use whole-grain flour). In a large bowl, mix the oats with the baking powder and baking soda. Mix the wet ingredients into the dry ingredients until just combined. Fold in the mix-ins (if using). Spoon about ¼ cup batter into each muffin cup and bake for 30 minutes, or until a toothpick inserted into the center comes out clean.

The orange creates a very moist base, so the muffins may take longer than 30 minutes, depending on how heavy your muffin tin is. Store the muffins in the fridge or freezer, because they are so moist. If you plan to keep them frozen, you can easily double the batch for a full dozen.

Per Serving: Calories: 287; Protein: 8g; Total fat: 12g; Carbohydrates: 41g; Fiber: 6g

08. Tortilla Breakfast Casserole

PREP: 20 MINUTES • COOK TIME: 20 MINUTES • TOTAL:40 MINUTES SERVES: 6

Ingredients

Nonstick cooking spray

1 recipe Tofu-Spinach Scramble

1 (14-ounce) can black beans, rinsed and drained

¼ cup nutritional yeast

2 teaspoons hot sauce

10 small corn tortillas

½ cup shredded vegan Cheddar or pepper Jack cheese, divided

Directions

Preparing the Ingredients.

Preheat the oven to 350°F.

Coat a 9-by-9-inch baking pan with cooking spray.

In a large bowl, combine the tofu scramble with the black beans, nutritional yeast, and hot sauce. Set aside.

In the bottom of the baking pan, place 5 corn tortillas. Spread half of the tofu and bean mixture over the tortillas. Spread ¼ cup of cheese over the top. Layer the remaining 5 tortillas over the top of the cheese. Spread the remainder of the tofu and bean mixture over the tortillas. Spread the remaining ¼ cup of cheese over the top.

Bake for 20 minutes. Divide evenly among 6 single-serving containers. Let cool before sealing the lids. Place the containers in the refrigerator for up to 5 days.

If you want to keep the casserole intact in the freezer, consider baking it in a disposable pan. Once cool, simply cover with foil and freeze.

Per Serving: Calories: 323; Protein: 27g; Carbohydrates: 60g; Fiber: 10g

09. **Savory Pancakes**

PREP: 10 MINUTES • COOK TIME: 15
MINUTES • TOTAL: 25 MINUTES
SERVES: 4

Ingredients

1 cup whole-wheat flour

1 teaspoon garlic salt

1 teaspoon onion powder

½ teaspoon baking soda

¼ teaspoon salt

1 cup lightly pressed, crumbled soft or firm
tofu

⅓ cup unsweetened plant-based milk

¼ cup lemon juice (about 2 small lemons)

2 tablespoons extra-virgin olive oil

½ cup finely chopped mushrooms

½ cup finely chopped onion

2 cups tightly packed greens (arugula, spinach,
or baby kale work great)

Nonstick cooking spray

Directions

Preparing the Ingredients.

In a large bowl, combine the flour, garlic salt, onion powder, baking soda, and salt. Mix well. In a blender, combine the tofu, plant-based milk, lemon juice, and olive oil. Purée on high speed for 30 seconds.

Pour the contents of the blender into the bowl of dry ingredients and whisk until combined well. Fold in the mushrooms, onion, and greens.

Spray a large skillet or griddle pan with nonstick cooking spray and set over medium-high heat. Reduce the heat to medium and add ½ cup of batter per pancake. Cook on both sides for about 3 minutes, or until set. After flipping, press down on the cooked side of the pancake with a spatula to flatten out the pancake. Repeat until the batter is gone. Divide the cooked pancakes among 4 single-serving containers. Let cool before sealing the lids.

Place the airtight storage containers in the refrigerator for up to 4 days. To reheat, microwave for 1½ to 2 minutes. To freeze, place the pancakes on a parchment paper-lined baking sheet in a single layer. If there's more than one layer, place another piece of parchment paper over the pancakes and place the second layer on top. Place the baking sheet in the freezer for 2 to 4 hours. Transfer the frozen pancakes to a freezer-safe bag (cut the parchment paper and place a small piece between each pancake). To thaw, refrigerate overnight. Preheat an oven or toaster oven to 350°F. Place the pancakes on a parchment paper-lined baking sheet and bake for 10 to 15 minutes, or stack the pancakes on a plate and microwave for 2 to 3 minutes.

Per Serving: Calories: 246; Protein: 10g; Total fat: 11g; Carbohydrates: 30g; Fiber: 3g

10. **Tropi-Kale Breeze**

PREP: 5 MINUTES • COOK TIME: 0MINUTES • TOTAL:5 MINUTES
SERVES: 4

Ingredients

1 cup chopped pineapple (frozen or fresh)

1 cup chopped mango (frozen or fresh)

½ to 1 cup chopped kale

½ avocado

½ cup coconut milk

1 cup of water, or coconut water

1 teaspoon matcha green tea powder (optional)

Directions

Preparing the Ingredients.

Pour everything in a blender until smooth, adding more water (or coconut milk) if needed.

Per Serving: Calories: 566; Protein: 8g; Total fat: 36g; Saturated fat: 1g; Carbohydrates: 66g; Fiber: 12g

11. **Blueberry Oatmeal Breakfast Bars**

PREP: 10 MINUTES • COOK TIME: 40 MINUTES • TOTAL:50 MINUTES SERVES: 12

Ingredients

2 cups uncooked rolled oats

2 cups all-purpose flour

1½ cups dark-brown sugar

1½ teaspoons baking soda

½ teaspoon sea salt

½ teaspoon ground cinnamon

1 cup vegan butter, melted

4 cups blueberries, fresh or frozen

¼ cup organic cane sugar

2 tablespoons cornstarch

Directions

Preparing the Ingredients.

Preheat the oven to 375°F. Lightly grease a 9-by-13-inch baking dish.

In a large bowl, combine the oats, flour, sugar, baking soda, salt, and cinnamon. Add the butter and mix until well incorporated and crumbly.

In a separate large bowl, combine the blueberries, cane sugar, and cornstarch, mixing until the blueberries are evenly coated. Press 3 cups of the oatmeal mixture into the prepared baking pan. Spread the blueberry mixture on top and crumble the remaining oatmeal mixture over the blueberries.
Bake for 40 minutes.
Remove from the oven and let cool completely before cutting into bars.

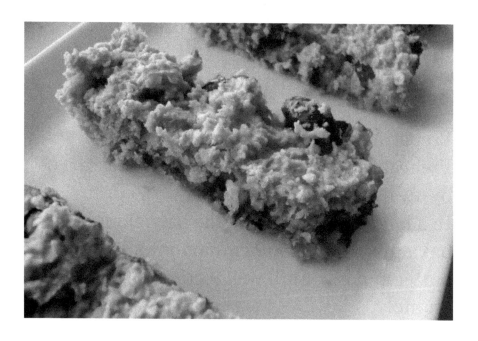

12. Quinoa Applesauce Muffins

PREP: 10 MINUTES • COOK TIME: 15 MINUTES • TOTAL: 25 MINUTES SERVES: 5

2 tablespoons coconut oil or margarine, melted, plus more for coating the muffin tin

¼ cup ground flaxseed

½ cup water

2 cups unsweetened applesauce

½ cup brown sugar

1 teaspoon apple cider vinegar

2½ cups whole-grain flour

1½ cups cooked quinoa

2 teaspoons baking soda

Pinch salt

½ cup dried cranberries or raisins

Preparing the Ingredients.

Preheat the oven to 400°F.

Coat a muffin tin with coconut oil, line with paper muffin cups, or use a nonstick tin. In a large bowl, stir together the flaxseed and water. Add the applesauce, sugar, coconut oil, and vinegar. Stir to combine. Add the flour, quinoa, baking soda, and salt, stirring until just combined. Gently fold in the cranberries without stirring too much. Scoop the muffin mixture into the prepared tin, about ⅓ cup for each muffin.

Bake for 15 to 20 minutes, until slightly browned on top and springy to the touch. Let cool for about 10 minutes. Run a dinner knife around the inside of each cup to loosen, then tilt the muffins on their sides in the muffin wells so air gets underneath. These keep in an airtight container in the refrigerator for up to 1 week or in the freezer indefinitely.

Per Serving (1 muffin): Calories: 387; Protein: 7g; Total fat: 5g; Saturated fat: 2g; Carbohydrates: 57g; Fiber: 8g

LUNCH

01.   Pad Thai Bowl

PREP: 10 MINUTES • COOK TIME: 10
MINUTES • TOTAL: 20 MINUTES
SERVES: 2

Ingredients

7 ounces brown rice noodles

1 teaspoon olive oil, or 1 tablespoon vegetable
broth or water

2 carrots, peeled or scrubbed, and julienned

1 cup thinly sliced napa cabbage, or red
cabbage

1 red bell pepper, seeded and thinly sliced

2 scallions, finely chopped

2 to 3 tablespoons fresh mint, finely chopped

1 cup bean sprouts

¼ cup Peanut Sauce

¼ cup fresh cilantro, finely chopped

2 tablespoons roasted peanuts, chopped

Fresh lime wedges

Directions

Preparing the Ingredients.

Put the rice noodles in a large bowl or pot, and cover with boiling water. Let sit until they soften, about 10 minutes. Rinse, drain, and set aside to cool. Heat the oil in a large skillet to medium-high, and sauté the carrots, cabbage, and bell pepper until softened, 7 to 8 minutes. Toss in the scallions, mint, and bean sprouts and cook for just a minute or two, then remove from the heat.

Toss the noodles with the vegetables, and mix in the Peanut Sauce. Transfer to bowls, and sprinkle with cilantro and peanuts. Serve with a lime wedge to squeeze onto the dish for a flavor boost.

Per Serving: Calories: 660; Total fat: 19g; Carbs: 110g; Fiber: 10g; Protein: 15g

Green Pea Risotto

PREP: 5 MINUTES • COOK TIME: 35
MINUTES • TOTAL: 40 MINUTES
SERVES: 4

Ingredients

1 teaspoon vegan butter

4 teaspoons minced garlic (about 4 cloves)

1 cup Arborio rice

2 cups vegetable broth (try a no-chicken broth
for a richer flavor)

¼ teaspoon salt

2 tablespoons nutritional yeast

3 tablespoons lemon juice (about 1½ small
lemons)

2 cups fresh, canned, or frozen (thawed) green
peas

¼ to ½ teaspoon freshly ground black pepper,
to taste

Directions

Preparing the Ingredients.

In a large skillet over medium-high heat, heat
the vegan butter.

Add the garlic and sauté for about 3 minutes.

Add the rice, broth, and salt, and stir to combine well.

Bring to boil. Reduce the heat to low and simmer for about 30 minutes until the broth is absorbed and the rice is tender. Stir in the nutritional yeast and lemon juice.

Gently fold in the peas. Taste before seasoning with the pepper.

Divide the risotto evenly among 4 single-serving containers. Let cool before sealing the lids.

Place the containers in the refrigerator for up to 5 days.

Per Serving: Calories: 144; Fat: 2g; Protein: 10g; Carbohydrates: 24g; Fiber: 7g; Sugar: 5g; Sodium: 273mg

03. **Caramelized Onion And Beet Salad**

PREP: 10 MINUTES • COOK TIME: 40
MINUTES • TOTAL: 50 MINUTES
SERVES: 4

Ingredients

3 medium golden beets

2 cups sliced sweet or Vidalia onions

1 teaspoon extra-virgin olive oil or no-beef
broth

Pinch baking soda

¼ to ½ teaspoon salt, to taste

2 tablespoons unseasoned rice vinegar, white
wine vinegar, or balsamic vinegar

Directions

Preparing the Ingredients.

Cut the greens off the beets, and scrub the
beets.

In a large pot, place a steamer basket and fill
the pot with 2 inches of water.

Add the beets, bring to a boil, then reduce the
heat to medium, cover, and steam for about 35
minutes, until you can easily pierce the middle
of the beets with a knife.

Meanwhile, in a large, dry skillet over medium heat, sauté the onions for 5 minutes, stirring frequently.

Add the olive oil and baking soda, and continuing cooking for 5 more minutes, stirring frequently. Stir in the salt to taste before removing it from the heat. Transfer to a large bowl and set aside.

When the beets have cooked through, drain and cool until easy to handle. Rub the beets in a paper towel to easily remove the skins. Cut into wedges, and transfer to the bowl with the onions. Drizzle the vinegar over everything and toss well.

Divide the beets evenly among 4 wide-mouth jars or storage containers. Let cool before sealing the lids.

Per Serving: Calories: 104; Fat: 2g; Protein: 3g; Carbohydrates: 20g; Fiber: 4g; Sugar: 14g; Sodium: 303mg

04. Grilled Portobello with Mashed Potatoes and Green Beans

PREP: 20 MINUTES • COOK TIME: 40 MINUTES • TOTAL: 60 MINUTES SERVES: 4

Ingredients

FOR THE GRILLED PORTOBELLOS

4 large portobello mushrooms

1 teaspoon olive oil

Pinch sea salt

FOR THE MASHED POTATOES

6 large potatoes, scrubbed or peeled, and chopped

3 to 4 garlic cloves, minced

½ teaspoon olive oil

½ cup non-dairy milk

2 tablespoons coconut oil (optional)

2 tablespoons nutritional yeast (optional)

Pinch sea salt

FOR THE GREEN BEANS

2 cups green beans, cut into 1-inch pieces

2 to 3 teaspoons coconut oil

Pinch sea salt

1 to 2 tablespoons nutritional yeast (optional)

TO MAKE THE GRILLED PORTOBELLOS

Preheat the grill to medium, or the oven to 350°F.

Take the stems out of the mushrooms.

Wipe the caps clean with a damp paper towel, then dry them. Spray the caps with a bit of olive oil, or put some oil in your hand and rub it over the mushrooms.

Rub the oil onto the top and bottom of each mushroom, then sprinkle them with a bit of salt on top and bottom.

Put the bottom side facing up on a baking sheet in the oven, or straight on the grill.

They'll take about 30 minutes in the oven, or 20 minutes on the grill. Wait until they're soft and wrinkling around the edges. If you keep the bottom up, all the delicious mushroom juice will pool in the cap. Then at the very end, you can flip them over to drain the juice. If you like it, you can drizzle it over the mashed potatoes.

Boil the chopped potatoes in lightly salted water for about 20 minutes, until soft. While they're cooking, sauté the garlic in the olive oil, or bake them whole in a 350°F oven for 10 minutes, then squeeze out the flesh. Drain the potatoes, reserving about ½ cup water to mash them. In a large bowl, mash the potatoes with a little bit of the reserved water, the cooked garlic, milk, coconut oil (if using), nutritional yeast (if using), and salt to taste. Add more water, a little at a time, if needed, to get the texture
you want. If you use an immersion blender or beater to purée them, you'll have some extra-creamy potatoes.

TO MAKE THE GREEN BEAN

Heat a medium pot with a small amount of water to boil, then steam the green beans by either putting them directly in the pot or in a steaming basket.
Once they're slightly soft and vibrantly green, 7 to 8 minutes, take them off the heat and toss them with the oil, salt, and nutritional yeast (if using).

Per Serving: Calories: 263; Total fat: 7g; Carbs: 43g; Fiber: 7g; Protein: 10g

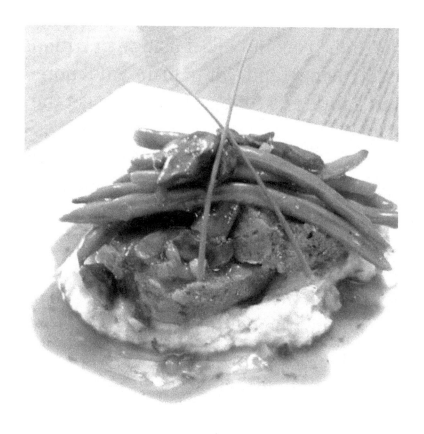

05

Italian Lentils

PREP: 5 MINUTES • COOK TIME: 40 MINUTES • TOTAL: 45 MINUTES SERVES: 6

Ingredients

5 cups water

2¼ cups dry French or brown lentils, rinsed and drained

3 teaspoons minced garlic (about 3 cloves)

1 bay leaf

½ teaspoon dried basil

½ teaspoon dried oregano

½ teaspoon dried rosemary

½ teaspoon dried thyme

Directions

Preparing the Ingredients.

In a large pot, combine the water, lentils, garlic, bay leaf, basil, oregano, rosemary, and thyme. Bring to a boil. Reduce the heat to low, cover, and simmer for 25 to 40 minutes, until tender, stirring occasionally. Drain any excess cooking liquid.

Transfer to a container, or scoop 1 cup of lentils into each of 6 storage containers. Let cool before sealing the lids.

Place the containers in the refrigerator for up to 5 days.

Per Serving (1 cup): Calories: 257; Fat: 1g; Protein: 19g; Carbohydrates: 44g; Fiber: 22g; Sugar: 2g; Sodium: 5mg

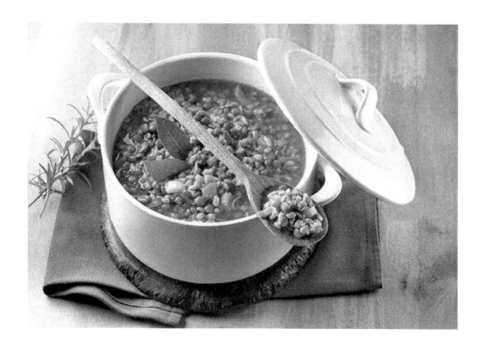

06

Roasted Cauliflower Tacos

PREP: 10 MINUTES • COOK TIME: 30
MINUTES • TOTAL: 40 MINUTES
SERVES: 8 TACOS

Ingredients

FOR THE ROASTED CAULIFLOWER

1 head cauliflower, cut into bite-size pieces

1 tablespoon olive oil (optional)

2 tablespoons whole-grain flour

2 tablespoons nutritional yeast

1 to 2 teaspoons smoked paprika

½ to 1 teaspoon chili powder

Pinch sea salt

FOR THE TACOS

2 cups shredded lettuce

2 cups cherry tomatoes, quartered

2 carrots, scrubbed or peeled, and grated

½ cup Fresh Mango Salsa

½ cup *Guacamole*

8 small whole-grain or corn tortillas

1 lime, cut into 8 wedges

Directions

TO MAKE THE ROASTED CAULIFLOWER
Preheat the oven to 350°F. Lightly grease a large rectangular baking sheet with olive oil, or line it with parchment paper. In a large bowl, toss the cauliflower pieces with oil (if using), or just rinse them so they're wet. The idea is to get the seasonings to stick. In a smaller bowl, mix together the flour, nutritional yeast, paprika, chili powder, and salt.
Add the seasonings to the cauliflower, and mix it around with your hands to thoroughly coat. Spread the cauliflower on the baking sheet, and roast for 20 to 30 minutes, or until softened.

TO MAKE THE TACOS.
Prep the veggies, salsa, and guacamole while the cauliflower is roasting. Once the cauliflower is cooked, heat the tortillas for just a few minutes in the oven or in a small skillet. Set everything out on the table, and assemble your tacos as you go. Give a squeeze of fresh lime just before eating.

Per Serving (1 taco): Calories: 198; Total fat: 6g; Carbs: 32g; Fiber: 6g; Protein: 7g

07

White Bean Burgers

PREP: 10 MINUTES • COOK TIME: 10
MINUTES • TOTAL: 20 MINUTES
SERVES: 4

Ingredients

1 tablespoon olive oil, plus more for coating
the baking sheet

¼ cup couscous

¼ cup boiling water

1 (15-ounce) can white beans, drained and
rinsed

2 tablespoons balsamic vinegar

2 tablespoons chopped sun-dried tomatoes or
olives

½ teaspoon garlic powder or 1 garlic clove,
finely minced

½ teaspoon salt

4 burger buns

Lettuce leaves, for serving

Tomato slices, for serving

Condiments of choice, such as ketchup, olive
tapenade, *Creamy Tahini Dressing*, and/or
Spinach Pesto

Directions

Preparing the Ingredients.

If baking, preheat the oven to 350°F.

1. Coat a rimmed baking sheet with olive oil or line it with parchment paper or a silicone mat. In a medium heat-proof bowl, combine the couscous and boiling water.

2. Cover and set aside for about 5 minutes. Once the couscous is soft and the water is absorbed, fluff it with a fork. Add the beans, and mash them to a chunky texture. Add the vinegar, olive oil, sun-dried tomatoes, garlic powder, and salt; stir until combined but still a bit chunky. Divide the mixture into 4 portions, and shape each into a patty. Put the patties on the prepared baking sheet, and bake for 25 to 30 minutes, until slightly crispy on the edges. Alternatively, heat some olive oil in a large skillet over medium heat, then add the patties, making sure each has oil under it.

3. Fry for about 5 minutes, until the bottoms are browned. Flip, adding more oil as needed, and fry for about 5 minutes more. Serve the burgers on buns with lettuce, tomato, and your choice of condiments.

08. **Loaded Black Bean Pizza**

PREP: 10 MINUTES • COOK TIME: 20 MINUTES • TOTAL: 30 MINUTES SERVES: 2 SMALL PIZZAS

Ingredients

2 prebaked pizza crusts

½ cup Spicy Black Bean Dip

1 tomato, thinly sliced

Pinch freshly ground black pepper

1 carrot, grated

Pinch sea salt

1 red onion, thinly sliced

1 avocado, sliced

 Preheat the oven to 400°F.

Directions

Preparing the Ingredients.

Lay the two crusts out on a large baking sheet. Spread half the Spicy Black Bean Dip on each pizza crust.

Then layer on the tomato slices with a pinch pepper if you like. Sprinkle the grated carrot with the sea salt and lightly massage it in with your hands.

Spread the carrot on top of the tomato, then add the onion.

Pop the pizzas in the oven for 10 to 20 minutes, or until they're done to your taste.

Top the cooked pizzas with sliced avocado and another sprinkle of pepper.

Per Serving (1 pizza) Calories: 379; Total fat: 13g; Carbs: 59g; Fiber: 15g; Protein: 13g

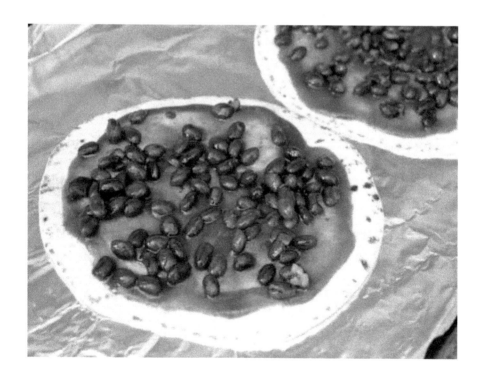

09. Curried Mango Chickpea Wrap

PREP: 15 MINUTES • COOK TIME: 0 MINUTES • TOTAL: 15 MINUTES SERVES: 3

Ingredients

3 tablespoons tahini

Zest and juice of 1 lime

1 tablespoon curry powder

¼ teaspoon sea salt

3 to 4 tablespoons water

1 (14-ounce) can chickpeas, rinsed and drained, or 1½ cups cooked

1 cup diced mango

1 red bell pepper, seeded and diced small

½ cup fresh cilantro, chopped

3 large whole-grain wraps

1 to 2 cups shredded green leaf lettuce

Directions

Preparing the Ingredients.

In a medium bowl, whisk together the tahini, lime zest and juice, curry powder, and salt until the mixture is creamy and thick.

Add 3 to 4 tablespoons of water to thin it out a bit. Or you can process this all in a blender. The taste should be strong and salty, to flavor the whole salad.

Toss the chickpeas, mango, bell pepper, and cilantro with the tahini dressing. Spoon the salad down the center of the wraps, top with shredded lettuce, and then roll up and enjoy.

Per Serving (1 wrap): Calories: 437; Total fat: 8g; Carbs: 79g; Fiber: 12g; Protein: 15g

10. Mom's Creamy Broccoli and Rice Bake

PREP: 10 MINUTES • COOK TIME: 40 MINUTES • TOTAL: 50 MINUTES SERVES: 7

Ingredients

2 cups cooked brown rice

1 (12-ounce) bag frozen broccoli florets, chopped, or 2 cups chopped fresh broccoli florets

½ cup chopped onion

1 celery stalk, thinly sliced

1 batch Easy Cheese Sauce

Directions

Preparing the Ingredients.

Preheat the oven to 425°F.

In a large bowl, mix together the rice, broccoli, onion, celery, and cheese sauce. Transfer to a 2-quart or 8-inch-square baking dish.

Bake for 40 minutes, or until the top has started to brown slightly.

Serve.

11. GGB Bowl

PREP: 10 MINUTES • COOK TIME: 5
MINUTES • TOTAL: 15 MINUTES
SERVES: 2

Ingredients

2 teaspoons olive oil

1 cup cooked brown rice, quinoa, or your grain
of choice

1 (15-ounce) can chickpeas or your beans of
choice, rinsed and drained

1 bunch spinach or kale, stemmed and roughly
chopped

1 tablespoon soy sauce or gluten-free tamari

Sea salt

Black pepper

Directions

Preparing the Ingredients.

1. In a large skillet, heat the oil over medium
heat.

2. Add the rice, beans, and greens and stir
continuously until the greens have wilted and
everything is heated for 3 to 5 minutes. Drizzle
in the soy sauce, mix to combine, and season
with salt and pepper.

Ratatouille (Pressure cooker)

PREP: 15 MINUTES • PRESSURE: 6 MINUTES • TOTAL: 45 MINUTES • PRESSURE LEVEL: HIGH • RELEASE: NATURAL

SERVES 4-6

Ingredients

1 onion, diced

4 garlic cloves, minced

1 to 2 teaspoons olive oil

1 cup water

3 or 4 tomatoes, diced

1 eggplant, cubed

1 or 2 bell peppers, any color, seeded and chopped

1½ tablespoons dried herbes de Provence (or any mixture of dried basil, oregano, thyme, marjoram, and rosemary)

½ teaspoon salt

Freshly ground black pepper

Directions

Preparing the Ingredients. On your electric pressure cooker, select Sauté. Add the onion, garlic, and olive oil. Cook for 4 to 5 minutes, stirring occasionally until the onion is softened. Add the water, tomatoes, eggplant, bell peppers, and herbes de Provence. Cancel Sauté.

High pressure for 6 minutes. Close and lock the lid, and select High Pressure for 6 minutes. Pressure Release. Once the cooking time is complete, let the pressure release naturally, about 20 minutes. Unlock and remove the lid. Let cool for a few minutes, then season with salt and pepper.

Per serving: Calories: 101; Total fat: 2g; Protein: 4g; Sodium: 304mg; Fiber: 7g

13. Lemon and Thyme Couscous

PREP: 5 MINUTES • COOK TIME: 10 MINUTES • TOTAL: 15 MINUTES SERVES: 6

Ingredients

2¾ cups vegetable stock

Juice and zest of 1 lemon

2 tablespoons chopped fresh thyme

1½ cups couscous

¼ cup chopped fresh parsley

Sea salt

Freshly ground black pepper

Directions

Preparing the Ingredients.

1. In a medium pot, bring the vegetable stock, lemon juice, and thyme to a boil. Stir in the couscous, cover, and remove from the heat.

2. Allow sitting, covered until the couscous absorbs the liquid and softens about 5 minutes. Fluff with a fork. Stir in the lemon zest and parsley.

3. Season with salt and pepper. Serve hot.

14. **Sushi-Style Quinoa**

PREP: 2 MINUTES • COOK TIME: 25 MINUTES • TOTAL: 27 MINUTES SERVES: 4

Ingredients

2 cups water

1 cup dry quinoa, rinsed

¼ cup unseasoned rice vinegar

¼ cup mirin or white wine vinegar

Directions

Preparing the Ingredients.

In a large saucepan, bring the water to a boil. Add the quinoa to the boiling water, stir, cover, and reduce the heat to low. Simmer for 15 to 20 minutes, until the liquid is absorbed. Remove from the heat and let stand for 5 minutes.

Fluff with a fork. Add the vinegar and mirin, and stir to combine well.

Divide the quinoa evenly among 4 mason jars or single-serving containers. Let cool before sealing the lids.

Per Serving: Calories: 192; Fat: 3g; Protein: 6g; Carbohydrates: 34g; Fiber: 3g; Sugar: 4g; Sodium: 132mg

DINNER

Coconut and Curry Soup

PREP: 15 MINUTES • COOK TIME: 15
MINUTES • TOTAL: 30 MINUTES
SERVES: 4

Ingredients

1 tablespoon coconut oil

½ onion, thinly sliced

1 carrot, peeled and julienned

½ cup sliced shiitake mushrooms

3 garlic cloves, minced

One 14-ounce can coconut milk

1 cup vegetable stock

Juice from 1 lime, or 2 teaspoons lime juice

½ teaspoon sea salt

2 teaspoons curry powder

Directions

Preparing the Ingredients

1. In a large soup pot, heat the coconut oil
over medium-high heat until it shimmers. Add
the onion, carrot, and mushrooms and cook
until soft, about 7 minutes. Stir in the garlic
and cook until it is fragrant about 30 seconds.

2. Add the coconut milk, vegetable stock, lime juice, salt, and curry powder and heat through. Serve immediately.

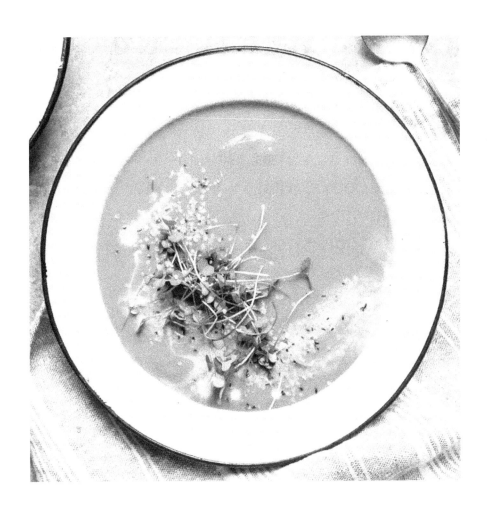

02. Split Pea Soup (Pressure Cooker)

PREP: 10 MINUTES • PRESSURE: 10 MINUTES • TOTAL: 45 MINUTES • PRESSURE LEVEL: HIGH • RELEASE: NATURAL

SERVES 6

Ingredients

3 or 4 carrots, scrubbed or peeled and chopped

1 large yellow onion, chopped

1 cup dried split green peas

3 cups water or unsalted vegetable broth

1 tablespoon tamari or soy sauce

2 to 3 teaspoons dried thyme or 1 teaspoon ground thyme

1 teaspoon onion powder

½ teaspoon garlic powder

Pinch freshly ground black pepper

¼ cup chopped sun-dried tomatoes or chopped pitted black olives

Salt

Directions

Preparing the Ingredients. Combine the carrots, onion, split peas, water, tamari, thyme, onion powder, garlic powder, and pepper in your pot.

High pressure for 10 minutes. Close and lock the lid, then select High Pressure and set the time for 10 minutes.

Pressure Release. Let the pressure release naturally, about 20 minutes. Unlock and remove the lid. Let cool for a few minutes and then purée the soup—transfer the soup (in batches, if necessary) to a countertop blender. Stir in the nutritional yeast (if using) and sun-dried tomatoes. Taste and season with salt.

Per Serving: Calories: 182; Protein: 12g; Total fat: 1g; Saturated fat: 11g; Carbohydrates: 26g; Fiber: 12g

03. **Weeknight Chickpea Tomato Soup**

PREP: 10 MINUTES • COOK TIME: 20 MINUTES • TOTAL: 30 MINUTES SERVES: 2

Ingredients

1 to 2 teaspoons olive oil, or vegetable broth

½ cup chopped onion

3 garlic cloves, minced

1 cup mushrooms, chopped

⅛ to ¼ teaspoon sea salt, divided

1 tablespoon dried basil

½ tablespoon dried oregano

1 to 2 tablespoons balsamic vinegar, or red wine

1 (19-ounce) can diced tomatoes

1 (14-ounce) can chickpeas, drained and rinsed, or 1½ cups cooked

2 cups water

1 to 2 cups chopped kale

Directions

Preparing the Ingredients.

In a large pot, warm the olive oil and sauté the onion, garlic, and mushrooms with a pinch salt until softened, 7 to 8 minutes. Add the basil and oregano and stir to mix. Then add the vinegar to deglaze the pan, using a wooden spoon to scrape all the browned, savory bits up from the bottom. Add the tomatoes and chickpeas. Stir to combine, adding enough water to get the consistency you want. Add the kale and the remaining salt. Cover and simmer for 5 to 15 minutes, until the kale is as soft as you like it.

This is delicious topped with a tablespoon of toasted walnuts and a sprinkle of nutritional yeast, or the Cheesy Sprinkle.

Per Serving: Calories: 343; Protein: 17g; Total fat: 9g; Carbohydrates: 61g; Fiber: 15g

04. **Minty Beet and Sweet Potato Soup**

PREP: 10 MINUTES • COOK TIME: 30 MINUTES • TOTAL: 40 MINUTES SERVES: 6

Ingredients

5 cups water, or salt-free vegetable broth (if salted, omit the sea salt below)

1 to 2 teaspoons olive oil, or vegetable broth

1 cup chopped onion

3 garlic cloves, minced

1 tablespoon thyme, fresh or dried

1 to 2 teaspoons paprika

2 cups peeled and chopped beets

2 cups peeled and chopped sweet potato

2 cups peeled and chopped parsnips

½ teaspoon sea salt

1 cup fresh mint, chopped

½ avocado, or 2 tablespoons nut or seed butter (optional)

2 tablespoons balsamic vinegar (optional)

2 tablespoons pumpkin seeds

Preparing the Ingredients.

In a large pot, boil the water. In another large pot, warm the olive oil and sauté the onion and garlic until softened about 5 minutes.

Add the thyme, paprika, beets, sweet potato, and parsnips, along with the boiling water and salt.

Cover and leave to gently boil for about 30 minutes, or until the vegetables are soft.

Set aside a little mint for a garnish and add the rest, along with the avocado (if using).

Stir until well combined.

Transfer the soup to a blender or use an immersion blender to purée, adding the balsamic vinegar (if using).

Serve topped with fresh mint and pumpkin seeds—and maybe chunks of the other half of the avocado, if you used it. This soup is perfect to make in big batches and keep in single-serving containers in the freezer for quick weeknight meals.

Per Serving: Calories: 156; Protein: 4g; Total fat: 4g; Carbohydrates: 31g; Fiber: 7g

05. Creamy Avocado-Dressed Kale Salad

PREP: 10 MINUTES • COOK TIME: 20 MINUTES • TOTAL: 30 MINUTES SERVES: 4

Ingredients

FOR THE DRESSING

1 avocado, peeled and pitted

1 tablespoon fresh lemon juice, or 1 teaspoon lemon juice concentrate and 2 teaspoons water

1 tablespoon fresh or dried dill

1 small garlic clove, pressed

1 scallion, chopped

Pinch sea salt

¼ cup water

FOR THE SALAD

8 large kale leaves

½ cup chopped green beans, raw or lightly steamed

1 cup cherry tomatoes, halved

1 bell pepper, chopped

2 scallions, chopped

2 cups cooked millet, or other cooked whole grain, such as quinoa or brown rice

Hummus (optional)

TO MAKE THE DRESSING

Put all the ingredients in a blender or food processor. Purée until smooth, then add water as necessary to get the consistency you're looking for in your dressing. Taste for seasoning, and add more salt if you need to.

TO MAKE THE SALAD

Chop the kale, removing the stems if you want your salad less bitter, and then massage the leaves with your fingers until it wilts and gets a bit moist about 2 minutes. You can use a pinch salt if you like to help it soften. Toss the kale with the green beans, cherry tomatoes, bell pepper, scallions, millet, and the dressing. Pile the salad onto plates, and top them off with a spoonful of hummus (if using).

Per Serving Calories: 225; Total fat: 7g; Carbs: 37g; Fiber: 7g; Protein: 7g

Miso Noodle Soup

PREP: 10 MINUTES • COOK TIME: 15
MINUTES • TOTAL: 25 MINUTES
SERVES: 4

Ingredients

7 ounces soba noodles (use 100% buckwheat
for gluten-free)
4 cups water
4 tablespoons miso
1 cup adzuki beans (cooked or canned),
drained and rinsed
2 tablespoons fresh cilantro, or basil, finely
chopped
2 scallions, thinly sliced

Directions

Preparing the Ingredients. Bring a large pot of
water to a boil, then add the soba noodles. Stir
them occasionally; they'll take about 5 minutes
to cook. Meanwhile, prepare the rest of the
soup by warming the water in a separate pot to
just below boiling, then remove it from heat.
Stir the miso into the water until it has
dissolved. Once the soba noodles are cooked,
drain them and rinse with hot water.

Add the cooked noodles, adzuki beans, cilantro, and scallions to the miso broth and serve.

Per Serving: Calories: 102; Protein: 11g; Total fat: 1g; Saturated fat: 11g; Carbohydrates: 18g; Fiber: 5g

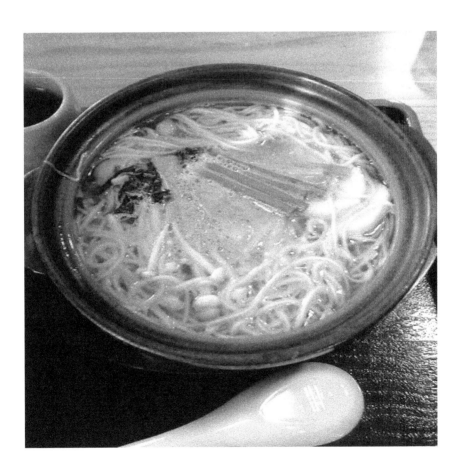

07. Creamy Butternut Squash Soup

PREP: 10 MINUTES • COOK TIME: 20 MINUTES • TOTAL: 30 MINUTES SERVES: 5

Ingredients

1 butternut squash (roughly 2 pounds), peeled, seeded, and cut into ½-inch cubes

1 red bell pepper, seeded and chopped

1 large onion, chopped

3 garlic cloves, minced

4 cups low-sodium vegetable broth

Juice of ½ lemon

2 tablespoons maple syrup

¾ teaspoon salt

¾ teaspoon black pepper

Directions

Preparing the Ingredients.

In a large stockpot, combine the squash, bell pepper, onion, garlic, and broth.

Mix well to combine, cover, and bring to a boil.

Reduce to a simmer and cook, covered, for 15 minutes, or until the squash is fork-tender. Add the lemon juice, maple syrup, salt, and pepper and stir well to combine.

Carefully transfer the soup to a blender. Remove the plug from the blender lid to allow steam to escape, hold a towel firmly over the hole in the lid, and blend until smooth.

Start at the lowest speed possible and increase gradually until the soup is completely smooth. Depending on your blender capacity, this might have to be done in two batches. (If you have an immersion blender, it would work great here.) Gently reheat over low heat to serve.

08. **Tabbouleh Salad**

PREP: 15 MINUTES • COOK TIME: 10 MINUTES • TOTAL: 25 MINUTES SERVES: 4

Ingredients

1 cup whole-wheat couscous

1 cup boiling water

Zest and juice of 1 lemon

1 garlic clove, pressed

Pinch of sea salt

1 tablespoon olive oil, or flaxseed oil (optional)

½ cucumber, diced small

1 tomato, diced small

1 cup fresh parsley, chopped

¼ cup fresh mint, finely chopped

2 scallions, finely chopped

4 tablespoons sunflower seeds (optional)

Directions

Preparing the Ingredients.

Put the couscous in a medium bowl, and cover with boiling water until all the grains are submerged. Cover the bowl with a plate or wrap. Set aside.

Put the lemon zest and juice in a large salad bowl, then stir in the garlic, salt, and olive oil (if using).

Put the cucumber, tomato, parsley, mint, and scallions in the bowl, and toss them to coat with the dressing. Take the plate off the couscous and fluff with a fork.

Add the cooked couscous to the vegetables, and toss to combine.

Serve topped with the sunflower seeds (if using).

Per Serving Calories: 304; Total fat: 11g; Carbs: 44g; Fiber: 6g; Protein: 10g

Cream of Mushroom Soup

PREP: 10 MINUTES • COOK TIME: 20
MINUTES • TOTAL: 30 MINUTES
SERVES: 2

Ingredients

1 to 2 teaspoons olive oil

1 onion, chopped

2 garlic cloves, minced

2 cups chopped mushrooms

Pinch salt

2 tablespoons whole-grain flour

1 teaspoon dried herbs

4 cups *Economical Vegetable Broth*, store-
bought broth, or water

1½ cups nondairy milk

Pinch freshly ground black pepper

Directions

Preparing the Ingredients.

Heat the olive oil in a large soup pot over
medium-high heat.

Add the onion, garlic, mushrooms, and salt.
Sauté for about 5 minutes, until softened.
Sprinkle the flour over the ingredients in the
pot and toss to combine.

Cook for 1 to 2 minutes more to toast the flour. Add the dried herbs, vegetable broth, milk, and pepper.

Turn the heat to low, and let the broth come to a simmer. (Don't bring to a full boil or the milk may separate.)

Cook for 10 minutes, until slightly thickened. Leftovers will keep in an airtight container for up to 1 week in the refrigerator or up to 1 month in the freezer.

Per Serving; Calories: 127; Protein: 4g; Total fat: 4g; Saturated fat: 0g; Carbohydrates: 21g; Fiber: 3g

10. **Glazed Curried Carrots**

PREP: 5 MINUTES • COOK TIME: 15
MINUTES • TOTAL: 20 MINUTES
SERVES: 6

Ingredients

1 pound carrots, peeled and thinly sliced

2 tablespoons olive oil

2 tablespoons curry powder

2 tablespoons pure maple syrup

Juice of ½ lemon

Sea salt

Freshly ground black pepper

Directions

Preparing the Ingredients.

Place the carrots in a large pot and cover with
water. Cook on medium-high heat until tender,
about 10 minutes. Drain the carrots and return
them to the pan over medium-low heat.

Stir in the olive oil, curry powder, maple syrup,
and lemon juice. Cook, stirring constantly,
until the liquid reduces, about 5 minutes.

Season with salt and pepper and serve
immediately.

Hot & Sour Tofu Soup

PREP: 40 MINUTES • COOK TIME: 15
MINUTES • TOTAL: 55MINUTES
SERVES: 3

Ingredients

6 to 7 ounces firm or extra-firm tofu

1 teaspoon olive oil

1 cup sliced mushrooms

1 cup finely chopped cabbage

1 garlic clove, minced

½-inch piece fresh ginger, peeled and minced

Salt

4 cups water or Economical Vegetable Broth

2 tablespoons rice vinegar or apple cider
vinegar

2 tablespoons soy sauce

1 teaspoon toasted sesame oil

1 teaspoon sugar

Pinch red pepper flakes

1 scallion, white and light green parts only,
chopped

Directions

Preparing the Ingredients.

Press your tofu before you start: Put it between several layers of paper towels and place a heavy pan or book (with a waterproof cover or protected with plastic wrap) on top. Let stand for 30 minutes. Discard the paper towels. Cut the tofu into ½-inch cubes.

In a large soup pot, heat the olive oil over medium-high heat.

Add the mushrooms, cabbage, garlic, ginger, and a pinch of salt. Sauté for 7 to 8 minutes, until the vegetables are softened.

Add the water, vinegar, soy sauce, sesame oil, sugar, red pepper flakes, and tofu.

Bring to a boil, then turn the heat to low.

Simmer the soup for 5 to 10 minutes.

Serve with the scallion sprinkled on top.

Leftovers will keep in an airtight container for up to 1 week in the refrigerator or up to 1 month in the freezer.

Per Serving (2 cups): Calories: 161; Protein: 13g; Total fat: 9g; Saturated fat: 1g; Carbohydrates: 10g; Fiber: 3g

12. **Rainbow Quinoa Salad**

PREP: 51 MINUTES • COOK TIME: 0
MINUTES • TOTAL: 15 MINUTES
SERVES: 6-8

Ingredients

3 tablespoons olive oil

Juice of 1½ lemons

1 teaspoon garlic powder

½ teaspoon dried oregano

1 bunch curly kale, stemmed and roughly
chopped

2 cups cooked tricolor quinoa

1 cup canned mandarin oranges in juice,
drained

1 cup diced yellow summer squash

1 red bell pepper, seeded and diced

½ red onion, thinly sliced

½ cup dried cranberries or cherries

½ cup slivered almonds

Directions

Preparing the Ingredients.

In a small bowl, whisk together the oil, lemon
juice, garlic powder, and oregano.

In a large bowl, toss the kale with the oil-lemon mixture until well coated. Add the quinoa, oranges, squash, bell pepper, and red onion and toss until all the ingredients are well combined. Divide among bowls or transfer to a large serving platter. Top with cranberries and almonds.

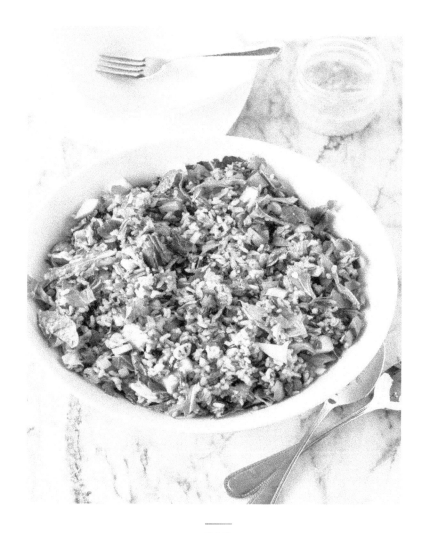

13. Eggplant Parmesan

PREP: 10 MINUTES • COOK TIME: 15
MINUTES • TOTAL: 25 MINUTES
SERVES: 1

Ingredients

¼ cup nondairy milk

¼ cup bread crumbs or panko

2 tablespoons nutritional yeast (optional)

¼ teaspoon salt

4 (¼-inch-thick) eggplant slices, peeled if
desired

1 tablespoon olive oil, plus more as needed

4 tablespoons Simple Homemade Tomato
Sauce

4 teaspoons Parm Sprinkle

Directions

Preparing the Ingredients.

1. Put the milk in a shallow bowl. In another
shallow bowl, stir together the bread crumbs,
nutritional yeast (if using), and salt.

2.   Dip one eggplant slice in the milk, making sure both sides get moistened. Dip it into the bread crumbs, flipping to coat both sides. Transfer to a plate and repeat to coat the remaining slices. Heat the olive oil in a large skillet over medium heat and add the breaded eggplant slices, making sure there is oil under each.

3.   Cook for 5 to 7 minutes, until browned. Flip, adding more oil as needed. Top each slice with 1 tablespoon tomato sauce and 1 teaspoon Parm Sprinkle. Cook for 5 to 7 minutes more. Per Serving Calories: 460; Protein: 23g; Total fat: 31g; Saturated fat: 4g; Carbohydrates: 31g; Fiber: 13g

DESSERT

01

Banana-Nut Bread Bars

PREP: 5 MINUTES • COOK TIME: 30
MINUTES • TOTAL: 5 MINUTES
SERVES: 9 BARS

Ingredients

Nonstick cooking spray (optional)

2 large ripe bananas

1 tablespoon maple syrup

½ teaspoon vanilla extract

2 cups old-fashioned rolled oats

½ teaspoons salt

¼ cup chopped walnuts

Directions

Preparing the Ingredients.

Preheat the oven to 350°F. Lightly coat a 9-by-9-inch baking pan with nonstick cooking spray (if using) or line with parchment paper for oil-free baking.

In a medium bowl, mash the bananas with a fork. Add the maple syrup and vanilla extract and mix well. Add the oats, salt, and walnuts, mixing well.

Transfer the batter to the baking pan and bake for 25 to 30 minutes, until the top is crispy. Cool completely before slicing into 9 bars. Transfer to an airtight storage container or a large plastic bag.

Per Serving (1 bar): Calories: 73; Fat: 1g; Protein: 2g; Carbohydrates: 15g; Fiber: 2g; Sugar: 5g; Sodium: 129mg

02

Apple Crumble

PREP: 20 MINUTES • COOK TIME: 25
MINUTES • TOTAL: 45 MINUTES
SERVES: 6

Ingredients

FOR THE FILLING

4 to 5 apples, cored and chopped (about 6
cups)

½ cup unsweetened applesauce, or ¼ cup
water

2 to 3 tablespoons unrefined sugar (coconut,
date, sucanat, maple syrup)

1 teaspoon ground cinnamon

Pinch sea salt

FOR THE CRUMBLE

2 tablespoons almond butter, or cashew or
sunflower seed butter

2 tablespoons maple syrup

1½ cups rolled oats

½ cup walnuts, finely chopped

½ teaspoon ground cinnamon

2 to 3 tablespoons unrefined granular sugar
(coconut, date, sucanat)

Directions

Preparing the Ingredients.

Preheat the oven to 350°F. Put the apples and applesauce in an 8-inch-square baking dish, and sprinkle with sugar, cinnamon, and salt. Toss to combine.

In a medium bowl, mix together the nut butter and maple syrup until smooth and creamy.

Add the oats, walnuts, cinnamon, and sugar and stir to coat, using your hands if necessary. (If you have a small food processor, pulse the oats and walnuts together before adding them to the mix.)

Sprinkle the topping over the apples, and put the dish in the oven.

Bake for 20 to 25 minutes, or until the fruit is soft and the topping is lightly browned.

Per Serving Calories: 356; Total fat: 17g; Carbs: 49g; Fiber: 7g; Protein: 7g

03

Cashew-Chocolate Truffles

PREP: 15 MINUTES • COOK TIME: 0
MINUTES • PLUS 1 HOUR TO SET
SERVES: 12 TRUFFLES

Ingredients

1 cup raw cashews, soaked in water overnight
¾ cup pitted dates
2 tablespoons coconut oil
1 cup unsweetened shredded coconut, divided
1 to 2 tablespoons cocoa powder, to taste

Directions

Preparing the Ingredients.

In a food processor, combine the cashews, dates, coconut oil, ½ cup of shredded coconut, and cocoa powder. Pulse until fully incorporated; it will resemble chunky cookie dough. Spread the remaining ½ cup of shredded coconut on a plate.

Form the mixture into tablespoon-size balls and roll on the plate to cover with the shredded coconut. Transfer to a parchment paper-lined plate or baking sheet. Repeat to make 12 truffles.

Place the truffles in the refrigerator for 1 hour to set. Transfer the truffles to a storage container or freezer-safe bag and seal.

Per Serving (1 truffle): Calories 238: Fat: 18g; Protein: 3g; Carbohydrates: 16g; Fiber: 4g; Sugar: 9g; Sodium: 9mg

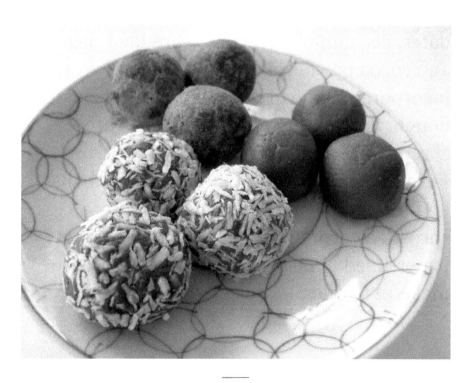

04. **Banana Chocolate Cupcakes**

PREP: 20 MINUTES • COOK TIME: 20 MINUTES • TOTAL: 40 MINUTES SERVES: 12 CUPCAKES

Ingredients

3 medium bananas

1 cup non-dairy milk

2 tablespoons almond butter

1 teaspoon apple cider vinegar

1 teaspoon pure vanilla extract

1¼ cups whole-grain flour

½ cup rolled oats

¼ cup coconut sugar (optional)

1 teaspoon baking powder

½ teaspoon baking soda

½ cup unsweetened cocoa powder

¼ cup chia seeds, or sesame seeds

Pinch sea salt

¼ cup dark chocolate chips, dried cranberries, or raisins (optional)

Directions

Preparing the Ingredients.

Preheat the oven to 350°F. Lightly grease the cups of two 6-cup muffin tins or line with paper muffin cups.

Put the bananas, milk, almond butter, vinegar, and vanilla in a blender and purée until smooth.

Or stir together in a large bowl until smooth and creamy.

Put the flour, oats, sugar (if using), baking powder, baking soda, cocoa powder, chia seeds, salt, and chocolate chips in another large bowl, and stir to combine. Mix together the wet and dry ingredients, stirring as little as possible. Spoon into muffin cups, and bake for 20 to 25 minutes. Take the cupcakes out of the oven and let them cool fully before taking them out of the muffin tins since they'll be very moist.

Per Serving (1 cupcake): Calories: 215; Total fat: 6g; Carbs: 39g; Fiber: 9g; Protein: 6g

05. **Minty Fruit Salad**

PREP: 15 MINUTES • COOK TIME: 5 MINUTES • TOTAL: 20 MINUTES SERVES: 4

Ingredients

¼ cup lemon juice (about 2 small lemons)

4 teaspoons maple syrup or agave syrup

2 cups chopped pineapple

2 cups chopped strawberries

2 cups raspberries

1 cup blueberries

8 fresh mint leaves

Directions

Preparing the Ingredients.

Beginning with 1 mason jar, add the ingredients in this order:

1 tablespoon of lemon juice, 1 teaspoon of maple syrup, ½ cup of pineapple, ½ cup of strawberries, ½ cup of raspberries, ¼ cup of blueberries, and 2 mint leaves.

Repeat to fill 3 more jars. Close the jars tightly with lids.

Place the airtight jars in the refrigerator for up to 3 days.

Per Serving: Calories: 138; Fat: 1g; Protein: 2g; Carbohydrates: 34g; Fiber: 8g; Sugar: 22g; Sodium: 6mg

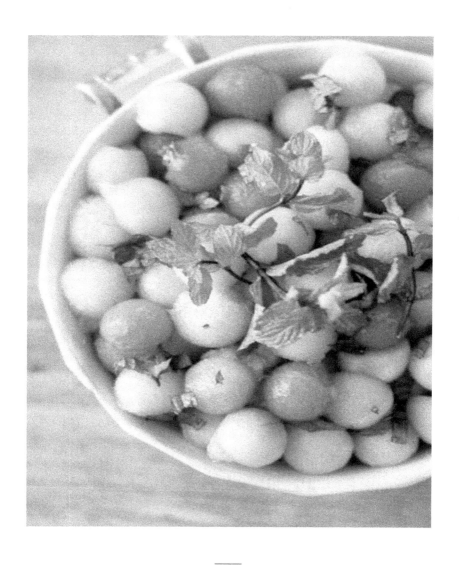

Mango Coconut Cream Pie

PREP: 20 MINUTES • CHILL TIME: 30
MINUTES • TOTAL: 50 MINUTES
SERVES: 8

Ingredients

FOR THE CRUST

½ cup rolled oats

1 cup cashews

1 cup soft pitted dates

FOR THE FILLING

1 cup canned coconut milk

½ cup water

2 large mangos, peeled and chopped, or about
2 cups frozen chunks

½ cup unsweetened shredded coconut

Directions

Preparing the Ingredients.

Put all the crust ingredients in a food
processor and pulse until it holds together. If
you don't have a food processor, chop
everything as finely as possible and use ½ cup
cashew or almond butter in place of half the
cashews. Press the mixture down firmly into
an 8-inch pie or springform pan.

Put the all filling ingredients in a blender and purée until smooth (about 1 minute). It should be very thick, so you may have to stop and stir until it's smooth.

Pour the filling into the crust, use a rubber spatula to smooth the top, and put the pie in the freezer until set, about 30 minutes. Once frozen, it should be set out for about 15 minutes to soften before serving.

Top with a batch of *Coconut Whipped Cream* scooped on top of the pie once it's set. Finish it off with a sprinkling of toasted shredded coconut.

Per Serving (1 slice): Calories: 427; Total fat: 28g; Carbs: 45g; Fiber: 6g; Protein: 8g

01. **Warm Quinoa Breakfast Bowl**

PREP: 5 MINUTES • COOK TIME: 0
MINUTES • TOTAL: 5 MINUTES
SERVES: 4

Ingredients

3 cups freshly cooked quinoa

1⅓ cups unsweetened soy or almond milk

2 bananas, sliced

1 cup raspberries

1 cup blueberries

½ cup chopped raw walnuts

¼ cup maple syrup

Directions

Preparing the Ingredients

Divide the ingredients among 4 bowls, starting with a base of ¾ cup quinoa, ⅓ cup milk, ½ banana, ¼ cup raspberries, ¼ cup blueberries, and 2 tablespoons walnuts.

Drizzle 1 tablespoon of maple syrup over the top of each bowl.

02. Not-Tuna Salad

PREP: 5 MINUTES • COOK TIME: 0
MINUTES • TOTAL: 5 MINUTES
SERVES: 4

Ingredients

1 (15.5-ounce) can chickpeas, drained and
rinsed

1 (14-ounce) can heart of palm, drained and
chopped

½ cup chopped yellow or white onion

½ cup diced celery

¼ cup vegan mayonnaise, plus more if needed

½ teaspoon salt

¼ teaspoon freshly ground black pepper

Directions

Preparing the Ingredients.

In a medium bowl, use a potato masher or fork
to roughly mash the chickpeas until chunky
and "shredded." Add the hearts of palm, onion,
celery, vegan mayonnaise, salt, and pepper.

Combine and add more mayonnaise, if necessary, for a creamy texture. Into each of 4 single-serving containers, place ¾ cup of salad. Seal the lids.

Per Serving: Calories: 214; Fat: 6g; Protein: 9g; Carbohydrates: 35g; Fiber: 8g; Sugar: 1g; Sodium: 765mg

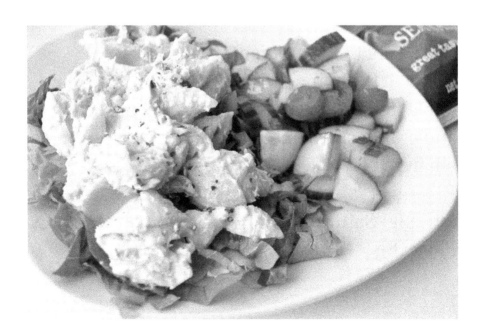

03. Apple-Sunflower Spinach Salad

PREP: 5 MINUTES • COOK TIME: 0 MINUTES • TOTAL: 5 MINUTES SERVES: 1

Ingredients

1 cup baby spinach

½ apple, cored and chopped

¼ red onion, thinly sliced (optional)

2 tablespoons sunflower seeds or Cinnamon-Lime Sunflower Seeds

2 tablespoons dried cranberries

2 tablespoons Raspberry Vinaigrette

Directions

Preparing the Ingredients.

Arrange the spinach on a plate. Top with the apple, red onion (if using), sunflower seeds, and cranberries, and drizzle with the vinaigrette.

Per Serving: Calories: 444; Protein: 7g; Total fat: 28g; Saturated fat: 3g; Carbohydrates: 53g; Fiber: 8g

Conclusion

Following the vegan diet has become extremely popular over the past decade. People switch for ethical and health reasons, and it is a great diet for people who are serious about getting healthy. But the one group of people that are still strongly judged about begin vegans are bodybuilders.

It has been a belief that the only way a person can gain muscle is by eating a bunch of lean poultry, dairy, and eggs. But the fact of the matter is, you can eat vegan and still gain muscle, and that's what this book is going to show you. Vegans come from all walks of life. They are of every nationality and every race. Being a vegan is more of a philosophy and lifestyle choice than it is an actual diet. The reasons for becoming a vegan could be to obtain better health, for environmental reasons, or due to the ethical concerns surrounding animal rights. Whatever the reasons may be for you, there is overwhelming evidence that shows how much healthier a vegan diet is for everyone, not just aspiring athletes. Some of the world's best athletes are vegan. This would not have been possible if a vegan diet had not met the needs of their bodies and increased their performance.

While many believe that a completely vegan diet is a new concept, it literally goes back almost until the dawn of human time.

Everyone is familiar with the Roman Gladiators. These athletes fought wild boars, lions, and each other in arenas cheered on by thousands of people. Discoveries in recent years have shown that the diet for most Gladiators was vegan. Even back then they were able to see the benefits that a vegan diet had on their performance while training and while fighting inside the arena.

A vegan diet has many health benefits. But is a vegan diet beneficial to an athlete?

Research has shown that diets that are high in foods from natural and unrefined sources play a great part in improving general health, immune systems, and cardio health.